Isometric Strength for Seniors

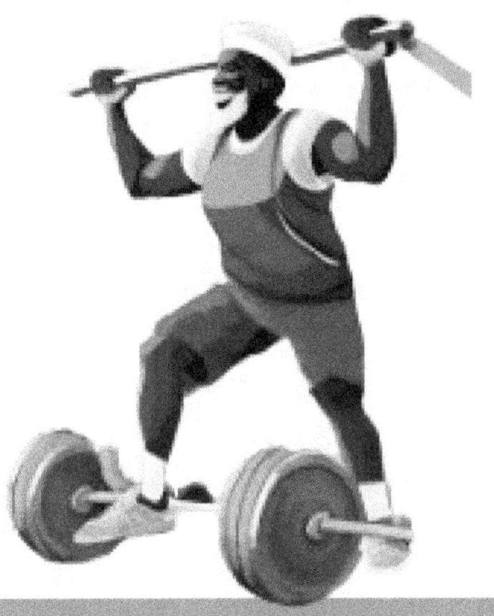

The Complete Guide To Safe And Effective Isometric Training For Older Adults To Improve Mobility, Flexibility, And Overall Health

Troy Vhodes

Table of Contents

Introduction

In the quiet moments of life's later chapters, where age graces us with wisdom and experience, there exists a profound desire for vitality, independence, and a renewed sense of well-being. It is within this sacred space that "Isometric Strength for Seniors" unfolds—a guide carefully crafted to resonate with the beating hearts and resilient spirits of those seeking not just exercise, but a transformative journey towards improved mobility, enhanced flexibility, and overall health.

Embrace the Journey: A Personal Odyssey

Let me share a personal revelation that ignited the creation of this comprehensive guide. Picture a moment where every movement felt like a challenge, where the shadows of stiffness and fatigue loomed large. It was within this struggle that isometric training emerged as a beacon of hope, transforming my own fitness journey. The metamorphosis was not just physical but a soul-stirring experience that laid the foundation for what you hold in your hands—a guide to rediscovering strength and vitality.

Unveiling the Canvas of Possibilities

Imagine a canvas where every stroke of isometric exercise paints a vibrant masterpiece of rejuvenation. In the pages ahead, you will witness the brushstrokes of improved mobility, the hues of enhanced flexibility, and the radiant colors of overall health. This is not just a workout guide; it is an invitation to step into a world where each pulse of energy becomes a celebration of life's enduring vitality.

Igniting the Spark: An Intriguing Revelation

Did you know that isometric training can not only sculpt the body but also elevate the spirit? In fact, studies reveal that seniors who embrace this transformative practice experience not just physical benefits but also a surge in mental well-being. The power of isometric strength is not merely confined to the body; it touches the essence of what it means to live life to the fullest.

In the Words of the Wise

As the echoes of strength resonate through time, let the words of revered athletes, trainers, and icons be your guiding force. "Isometric Strength for Seniors" is not just a guide; it is an embodiment of wisdom from those who have paved the way, testifying to the life-changing potential of this form of exercise.

Embark on the Journey with Purpose

Now, imagine standing at the threshold of a rejuvenated life. Can you envision the possibilities that lie ahead? "Isometric Strength for Seniors" is not just a guide; it is your passport to a realm of strength and vitality. In the chapters to come, we unravel the uniqueness of isometric training, delve into personal anecdotes, answer intriguing questions, and present you with a roadmap of big takeaways that will redefine your understanding of fitness.

Chapter 1
The Aging Body and Isometric Training
Exploring the Changes in Senior Muscles and Joints

Introduction:

Welcome to the foundational chapter of "Isometric Strength for Seniors," where we embark on an exploration of the intricate relationship between aging bodies and the transformative power of isometric training. In this chapter, we delve deep into the physiological changes that occur in senior muscles and joints, unraveling the narrative of how isometric training becomes not just an exercise routine but a key to unlocking vitality.

Understanding the Aging Process:

As time gracefully advances, our bodies undergo a natural evolution. Muscles, once spry and responsive, gradually encounter changes that can affect strength, flexibility, and overall functionality. Connective tissues lose some of their elasticity, and joints may experience a decrease in fluidity. Understanding this aging process is crucial for tailoring fitness practices to align with the body's evolving needs.

The Role of Isometric Training:

Enter isometric training—a beacon of hope in the landscape of aging. Isometric exercises, by nature, involve muscle contraction without joint movement.

This characteristic is particularly advantageous for seniors, as it minimizes stress on joints while effectively engaging muscles. Isometric training becomes a gentle yet potent ally in navigating the nuances of aging, offering a unique approach to preserving and enhancing muscular strength.

Muscular Changes and Isometric Solutions:

Loss of Muscle Mass (Sarcopenia):

Explanation: With age, the body may experience sarcopenia, the gradual loss of muscle mass. This can lead to reduced strength and increased vulnerability to injury.

Isometric Solution: Isometric exercises, with their static muscle contractions, stimulate muscle fibers effectively, promoting muscle retention and countering the effects of sarcopenia.

Joint Stiffness and Decreased Range of Motion:

Explanation: Joints may become stiffer over time, limiting the range of motion. This stiffness can impact daily activities and overall mobility.

Isometric Solution: Isometric exercises, by nature of their static nature, help improve joint stability without subjecting them to excessive movement. This contributes to enhanced flexibility and joint health.

Decline in Muscle Elasticity:

Explanation: Aging muscles may experience a decline in elasticity, affecting their ability to stretch and contract optimally.

Isometric Solution: Isometric holds, strategically incorporated into training, contribute to improved muscle elasticity, fostering a greater range of motion and flexibility.

The Synergy of Aging Gracefully with Isometric Strength:

As we conclude this chapter, envision the symbiotic dance between the aging body and the rejuvenating influence of isometric training. Each static contraction becomes a deliberate step towards preserving strength, enhancing flexibility, and fostering overall well-being. In the pages that follow, we'll delve deeper into the practical aspects of isometric exercises, ensuring that every movement aligns with the unique needs of seniors, crafting a journey towards not just fitness, but a vibrant and empowered existence.

Key Takeaways:
- Sarcopenia, joint stiffness, and reduced muscle elasticity are common challenges in aging bodies.
- Isometric training serves as a tailored solution, addressing these challenges with static muscle contractions.
- Isometric exercises contribute to muscle retention, improved joint stability, and enhanced flexibility, offering seniors a path to graceful aging.

How Isometric Training Addresses Age-Related Challenges

Introduction:

As we embark on this Chapter of "Isometric Strength for Seniors," we unravel the remarkable synergy between isometric training and the challenges posed by the inexorable march of time. Here, we explore how isometric exercises serve as a tailored response to age-related hurdles, becoming a beacon of resilience for the aging body.

The Uniqueness of Isometric Training:

Isometric training stands as a distinctive approach in the realm of fitness, and its uniqueness lies in its ability to directly confront and counter age-related challenges. Unlike dynamic exercises that involve joint movement, isometric training relies on static contractions, offering a gentler yet highly effective strategy for addressing the specific needs of seniors.

Mitigating Joint Stress:

One primary challenge seniors face is the wear and tear on joints, often resulting in discomfort and reduced mobility. Isometric exercises, with their static nature, minimize joint stress while still engaging muscles. This deliberate approach allows for strengthening without subjecting the joints to excessive movement, making isometric training a safe haven for those seeking relief from age-induced joint issues.

Counteracting Muscle Loss:

Sarcopenia, the age-related loss of muscle mass, can lead to a decline in strength and overall functionality. Isometric training becomes a stalwart ally in counteracting this muscle loss. The sustained contractions inherent in isometric exercises stimulate muscle fibers, promoting muscle retention and preventing the debilitating effects of sarcopenia.

Enhancing Joint Stability:

The static nature of isometric exercises proves invaluable in enhancing joint stability. For seniors grappling with joint stiffness or decreased range of motion, isometric training becomes a means to gently challenge and improve joint function without subjecting them to abrupt movements. This targeted approach fosters increased joint stability, contributing to overall mobility.

Improving Functional Strength:

Isometric exercises go beyond the superficial, addressing the very essence of functional strength. The static holds, strategically executed, target specific muscle groups that are crucial for daily activities. As a result, seniors find themselves not only gaining physical strength but also experiencing a renewed capacity to perform everyday tasks with greater ease and confidence.

Elevating Flexibility and Range of Motion:

Age can bring about a decline in muscle elasticity, limiting flexibility and range of motion. Isometric training, when integrated thoughtfully, serves as a remedy.

By promoting controlled stretching and contraction, isometric exercises contribute to improved muscle elasticity, enabling seniors to move more freely and comfortably.

Conclusion:
In the intricate dance between aging and isometric training, this Chapter illustrates the harmonious rhythm where challenges are met with purposeful resistance. Isometric exercises emerge not as a mere workout routine but as a tailored response, a guiding force that empowers seniors to navigate age-related hurdles with resilience and strength.

Key Takeaways:
- Isometric training, with its static contractions, minimizes stress on joints, providing relief for seniors with joint issues.
- Sustained muscle contractions in isometric exercises counteract the effects of sarcopenia, preserving and enhancing muscle mass.
- Isometric training fosters joint stability, addressing issues of stiffness and limited range of motion.
- Functional strength is improved through targeted isometric exercises, enhancing seniors' ability to perform daily activities.
- Isometric training contributes to the elevation of flexibility and range of motion, mitigating the decline in muscle elasticity associated with aging.

Chapter 2
Getting Started with Isometric Exercises
The Basics of Isometric Training

Introduction:

Welcome to the heart of "Isometric Strength for Seniors." In Chapter 2, we embark on a practical journey, laying the foundation for your isometric training experience. Here, we unravel the basics of isometric training, providing a step-by-step guide that ensures you not only understand the exercises but also execute them with confidence and precision.

The Essence of Isometric Training:

Before we dive into the exercises themselves, let's grasp the essence of isometric training. Unlike traditional exercises that involve dynamic movements, isometric training revolves around static contractions. This means that during an isometric exercise, your muscles contract without changing their length. This unique approach offers a wealth of benefits, especially for seniors looking to improve strength, mobility, and overall health.

Creating Your Isometric Space:

Before embarking on the exercises, it's crucial to designate a comfortable and safe space. Choose an area with ample room for movement and a supportive surface. Consider using a mat or non-slip surface to enhance stability during exercises. Creating a dedicated space ensures that you can focus on your training without distractions.

Starting with Isometric Holds:

The cornerstone of isometric training lies in the concept of holds. These are static contractions where you maintain a specific position for a set duration. Let's break down the basics of isometric holds:

Bodyweight Squat Hold:

Execution:

1. Stand with feet shoulder-width apart.

2. Lower your body into a squat position, keeping your back straight and knees aligned with your toes.

3. Hold the position for 20 seconds, gradually increasing the duration as you become more comfortable.

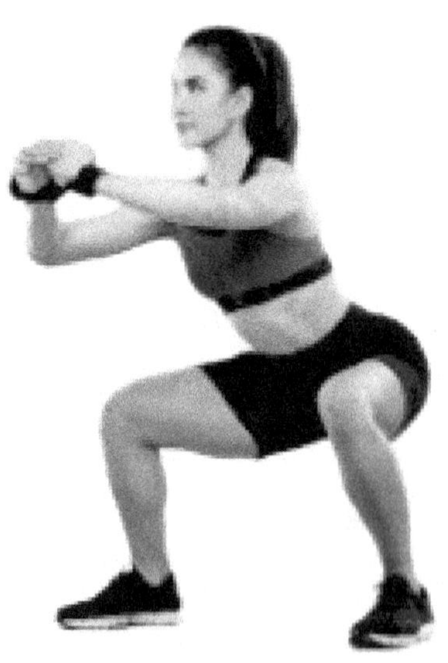

Execution:

1. Stand facing a wall with arms extended.

2. Perform a push-up against the wall, stopping midway and holding the position.

3. Hold for 15 seconds, focusing on engaging your chest and arm muscles.

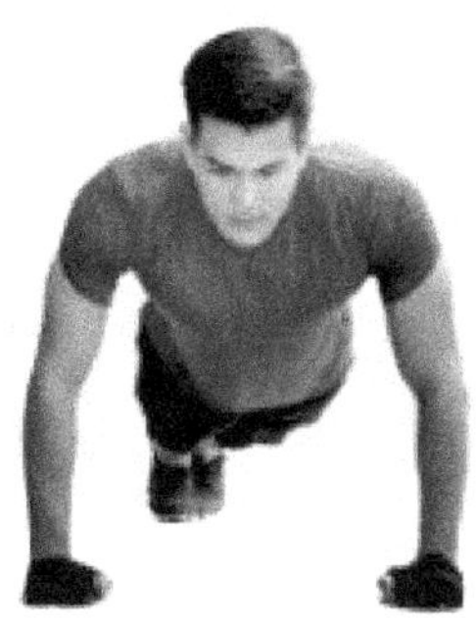

Incorporating Isometric Contractions into Everyday Activities:

Isometric exercises can seamlessly integrate into your daily routine. Let's explore how to infuse isometric contractions into everyday activities:

Isometric Leg Press while Seated:

Execution:

1. While sitting, place your hands on your thighs.

2. Attempt to press your hands and thighs together, engaging your leg muscles.

3. Hold the contraction for 15 seconds, gradually increasing the duration.

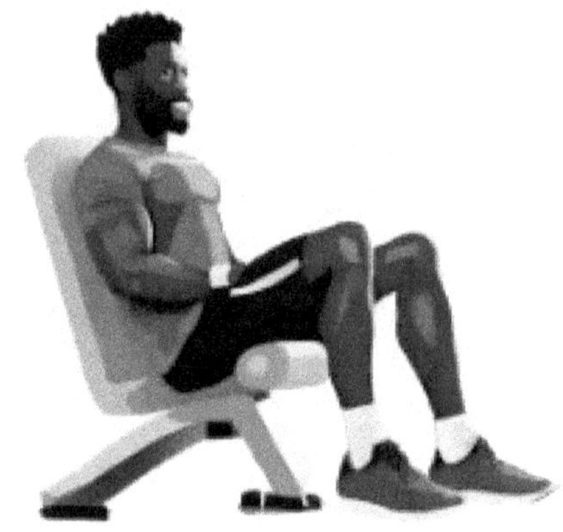

Desk Push:

Execution:

1. While sitting at a desk, place your palms on the surface.

2. Push against the desk, activating your chest and arm muscles.

3. Hold for 20 seconds, feeling the muscles engage.

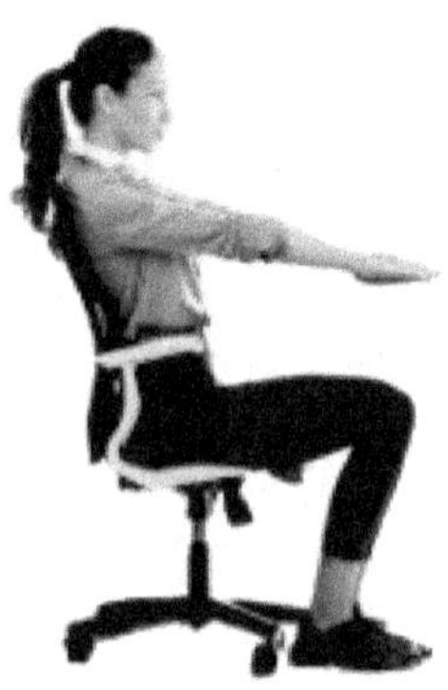

Assessing Your Current Fitness Level:
Understanding your current fitness level is crucial for tailoring isometric exercises to your specific needs. Before progressing further, take a moment to assess your strength, flexibility, and any existing limitations. This self-awareness will guide you in selecting appropriate exercises and customizing routines that align with your fitness journey.

Conclusion:

This chapter serves as the gateway to your isometric training odyssey. By mastering the basics of isometric holds and seamlessly incorporating contractions into your daily life, you lay the groundwork for a transformative experience. As you move forward, these foundational exercises will become the building blocks of a stronger, more resilient you.

Key Takeaways:

- Isometric training revolves around static contractions, offering unique benefits for seniors.
- Create a dedicated space for your isometric exercises, ensuring a comfortable and safe environment.
- Master the basics of isometric holds, including bodyweight squat holds and wall push-up holds.
- Infuse isometric contractions into everyday activities, seamlessly integrating them into your routine.
- Assess your current fitness level to customize isometric exercises based on your individual needs.

With this knowledge in hand, turn the page and let the practical journey of isometric training begin. Each hold, each contraction, becomes a step toward unlocking the full potential of your strength and mobility.

Assessing Your Current Fitness Level

Introduction:

Before embarking on any fitness journey, it's crucial to establish a starting point. Chapter 2.5 of "Isometric Strength for Seniors" guides you through the process of assessing your current fitness level. This self-awareness is fundamental for tailoring your isometric training experience to meet your individual needs and capabilities.

Understanding Your Strength:

Assessing your current strength is the first step in crafting a personalized isometric training plan. Consider the following:

Upper Body Strength:

Self-Assessment:

1. Perform a simple push-up against a wall or on a stable surface.

2. Note the ease or difficulty in completing the movement.

Lower Body Strength:

Self-Assessment:

1. Stand up and sit down from a chair without using your hands.

2. Take note of any challenges or discomfort.

Core Strength:

Self-Assessment:

1. Attempt a plank position, either on your hands or forearms.

2. Observe how long you can comfortably hold the plank.

Assessing Flexibility:

Flexibility is a key component of overall mobility. Evaluate your current flexibility with these simple assessments:

Shoulder Flexibility:

Self-Assessment:

1. Reach one arm behind your head and attempt to touch the middle of your upper back.
2. Note the range of motion and any tightness.

Lower Body Flexibility:

Self-Assessment:

1. While seated, extend one leg and reach toward your toes.
2. Evaluate the reach and any discomfort or restriction.

Identifying Limitations:

Understanding any existing limitations is crucial for designing a safe and effective isometric training plan. Consider the following:

Joint Limitations:

Self-Reflection:

1. Identify any joints that have limited range of motion or cause discomfort.
2. Consider past injuries or conditions that may impact your movements.

Self-Reflection:

1. Reflect on any health conditions or concerns that may affect your ability to engage in certain exercises.

2. Consider consulting with a healthcare professional for personalized guidance.

Conclusion:

As we conclude Chapter 2.5, remember that assessing your current fitness level is not a judgment but a roadmap for progress. By understanding your strengths, flexibility, and potential limitations, you empower yourself to tailor your isometric training experience to align with your unique needs. This self-awareness becomes the compass guiding you towards a stronger, more resilient you.

Key Takeaways:

- Evaluate upper body, lower body, and core strength to understand your current physical capabilities.
- Assess shoulder and lower body flexibility to gauge your range of motion.
- Identify any joint limitations or health considerations that may impact your training.
- Use this self-awareness to tailor isometric exercises to your individual needs and abilities.

With this self-assessment, you're equipped with the knowledge needed to navigate the isometric training journey with confidence. Turn the page, and let your personalized exploration of strength and mobility unfold.

Chapter 3
Safe and Effective Techniques for Seniors
Importance of Proper Form and Posture

Introduction:

Chapter 3 of "Isometric Strength for Seniors" delves into the paramount importance of safe and effective techniques when engaging in isometric training. For seniors, proper form and posture are not mere recommendations but the bedrock of a secure and fruitful fitness journey.

The Foundation of Proper Form:

Before delving into specific isometric exercises, let's first establish why proper form is foundational for seniors:

Injury Prevention:

Explanation:

1. Incorrect form can strain muscles and joints, leading to potential injuries.

2. Seniors, with their unique physical considerations, benefit greatly from injury prevention through proper form.

Maximizing Effectiveness:

Explanation:

1. Proper form ensures that the intended muscle groups are targeted during isometric exercises.

2. This maximizes the effectiveness of each movement, contributing to overall strength and mobility.

Understanding the Role of Posture:

Posture is not just about standing or sitting up straight; it influences the efficacy and safety of isometric exercises:

Spinal Alignment:

Explanation:

1. Maintaining a neutral spine during exercises prevents undue stress on the back.

2. This is particularly vital for seniors, considering the potential impact on spinal health.

Joint Alignment:

Explanation:

1. Proper posture ensures that joints are aligned correctly during exercises.

2. This alignment minimizes the risk of strain or discomfort, promoting a safer workout.

Achieving Proper Form and Posture:

Now that we recognize the importance of form and posture, let's explore practical steps to achieve them:

Mindful Movement:

Guidance:

1. Focus on each movement, ensuring a deliberate and controlled approach.

2. Mindful movement establishes a mind-body connection, reducing the likelihood of improper form.

Neutral Spine Awareness:

Guidance:

1. Emphasize a neutral spine, maintaining the natural curvature of the spine during exercises.

2. Engage core muscles to support the spine and enhance stability.

Joint Alignment Checks:

Guidance:

1. Regularly assess joint alignment, particularly during static holds.

2. Make adjustments as needed to ensure joints are in a safe and supported position.

Tailoring Techniques for Individual Needs:

Recognizing that every senior has unique considerations, the importance of tailoring techniques is highlighted:

Modifications for Comfort:

Guidance:

1. Explore modifications for exercises that may cause discomfort.

2. Personalize each movement to accommodate individual needs and limitations.

Gradual Progression:

Guidance:

1. Begin with simpler exercises and gradually progress to more advanced ones.

2. This incremental approach allows for the development of proper form over time.

Conclusion:

As we conclude Chapter 3, the significance of safe and effective techniques for seniors becomes evident. By embracing proper form and posture, you not only safeguard your well-being but also pave the way for a more impactful isometric training experience. This chapter serves as a guide, emphasizing that the journey towards strength and mobility should be as secure as it is empowering.

Key Takeaways:
- Proper form is essential for injury prevention and maximizing the effectiveness of isometric exercises.
- Posture influences spinal and joint alignment, impacting the safety and efficacy of workouts.
- Achieve proper form through mindful movement, neutral spine awareness, and regular joint alignment checks.
- Tailor techniques to individual needs with modifications and gradual progression.

Turn the page, carrying with you the understanding that the importance of form and posture is not a hurdle but a cornerstone of your isometric strength journey.

Adapting Isometric Exercises for Different Fitness Levels

Introduction:

In this Chapter of "Isometric Strength for Seniors," we embark on the journey of tailoring isometric exercises to meet the diverse needs of individuals at various fitness levels. Recognizing that each person has a unique starting point, this chapter delves into the art of adaptation, ensuring that isometric training remains accessible and beneficial for all.

Embracing Diversity in Fitness:

The fitness journey is as diverse as the individuals undertaking it. Understanding and embracing this diversity is crucial for fostering inclusivity in isometric training:

Varied Fitness Backgrounds:

Explanation:

1. Individuals may have varying levels of fitness experience.

2. Adapting isometric exercises ensures accessibility for both beginners and seasoned fitness enthusiasts.

Addressing Physical Limitations:

Explanation:

1. Different fitness levels may be accompanied by unique physical considerations.

2. Adaptations allow for customization, addressing limitations and ensuring safety.

Adapting for Beginners:

For those new to isometric training, creating a foundation of comfort and confidence is paramount:

Introduction to Basic Holds:

Guidance:

1. Begin with simple isometric holds, such as wall squats or chair sits.

2. Gradually increase hold durations as strength and familiarity grow.

Supportive Modifications:

Guidance:

1. Introduce modifications that provide additional support, such as using a stable surface for push-ups.

2. These modifications build strength progressively and instill confidence.

Catering to Intermediate Levels:

Individuals with moderate fitness backgrounds benefit from a balance of challenge and accessibility:

Incorporating Dynamic Elements:

Guidance:

1. Introduce dynamic elements within isometric exercises, adding controlled movements.

2. This progression enhances overall engagement and promotes strength development.

Gradual Intensity Increases:

Guidance:

1. Gradually increase the intensity of static holds and incorporate more advanced exercises.

2. This approach ensures a continuous challenge while respecting the individual's capabilities.

Challenging Advanced Participants:

For those well-versed in isometric training, the focus shifts to pushing boundaries safely:

Introducing Compound Movements:

Guidance:

1. Combine isometric exercises with dynamic, compound movements.

2. This advanced approach challenges multiple muscle groups simultaneously, promoting comprehensive strength.

Progressive Duration and Resistance:

Guidance:

1. Extend hold durations and introduce resistance to intensify workouts.

2. Progressive overload ensures ongoing development for advanced participants.

Personalization and Individual Progression:

The key to successful adaptation lies in personalization and allowing for individual progression:

Guidance:

1. Encourage participants to self-pace, tailoring workouts to their comfort and challenge levels.

2. This autonomy fosters a positive and empowering fitness experience.

Monitoring and Adjusting:

Guidance:

1. Regularly monitor individual progress and comfort levels.

2. Adjust exercises and intensity based on personal feedback to optimize effectiveness.

Conclusion:

This chapter encapsulates the spirit of inclusivity in isometric training, reminding us that fitness is a personal journey with diverse starting points. By adapting isometric exercises to different fitness levels, we ensure that everyone, regardless of experience, finds a path to strength, mobility, and overall well-being.

Key Takeaways:

- Embrace diversity in fitness backgrounds and physical limitations.
- Adapt isometric exercises for beginners with basic holds and supportive modifications.
- Cater to intermediate levels with dynamic elements and gradual intensity increases.
- Challenge advanced participants with compound movements and progressive duration/resistance.
- Prioritize personalization, self-pacing, and continuous monitoring for individual progression.

Chapter 4
Tailoring Isometric Routines to Your Needs
Customizing Workouts for Mobility Improvement

Introduction:

In Chapter 4 of "Isometric Strength for Seniors," we explore the art of customizing isometric routines to align with individual needs. This chapter focuses specifically on tailoring workouts for mobility improvement, a key aspect of enhancing overall well-being. Join us on this journey of personalization and empowerment.

The Significance of Mobility:

Before diving into customization, let's understand why mobility holds a pivotal role in the context of isometric training:

Freedom of Movement:

Explanation:

    1. Mobility refers to the ability to move freely and easily.

    2. Isometric routines tailored for mobility improvement contribute to a more fluid and unrestricted range of motion.

Explanation:

1. Improved mobility enhances functional independence in daily activities.

2. Customized isometric workouts address specific mobility concerns, fostering autonomy.

Identifying Mobility Goals:

Begin the customization process by identifying your personal mobility goals:

Range of Motion Targets:

Guidance:

1. Assess specific areas where you seek improved range of motion.

2. Tailor isometric exercises to target and enhance flexibility in these areas.

Daily Functionality:

Guidance:

1. Consider daily activities that may benefit from increased mobility.

2. Customize workouts to address the specific movements required for these activities.

Adapting Isometric Exercises:

Now, let's explore how to adapt isometric exercises to target and enhance mobility:

Joint-Specific Holds:

Guidance:

1. Identify joints requiring increased mobility.

2. Tailor holds that specifically target these joints, focusing on controlled stretches.

Dynamic Isometrics:

Guidance:

1. Introduce dynamic elements within isometric exercises.

2. This combination of static contractions and controlled movements enhances both strength and mobility.

Incorporating Progressive Challenges:

To continually improve mobility, it's essential to introduce progressive challenges:

Gradual Intensity Increase:

Guidance:

1. Gradually increase the intensity of isometric holds over time.

2. This progression ensures a consistent challenge, promoting continuous improvement.

Resistance Integration:

Guidance:

1. Integrate resistance, such as light weights or resistance bands, into isometric exercises.

2. Resistance adds an extra dimension, fostering both strength and increased mobility.

Personalization for Individual Needs:

Personalization is the key to effective customization. Consider individual needs when tailoring isometric routines for mobility:

Addressing Specific Concerns:

Guidance:

1. Tailor routines to address specific mobility concerns or limitations.

2. This individualized approach ensures targeted improvement.

Consistent Feedback Loop:

Guidance:

1. Encourage consistent feedback on comfort levels and perceived improvement.

2. Adjust routines based on individual responses, creating a dynamic and responsive training plan.

Conclusion:

As this chapter concludes, the emphasis on personalization and mobility improvement remains at the forefront. By tailoring isometric routines to your specific needs, focusing on mobility enhancement, you embark on a transformative journey towards a more flexible, capable, and empowered self.

Key Takeaways:

- Mobility improvement is a crucial aspect of isometric training for overall well-being.
- Identify specific mobility goals and areas requiring increased range of motion.

- Adapt isometric exercises with joint-specific holds and dynamic elements.
- Introduce progressive challenges, including gradual intensity increases and resistance integration.
- Personalize routines based on individual needs and provide a consistent feedback loop for continuous improvement.

Targeting Flexibility and Joint Health Through Isometric Training

Introduction:

In this Chapter of "Isometric Strength for Seniors," we embark on a specialized exploration of how isometric training becomes a dynamic tool for targeting flexibility and promoting joint health. This chapter delves into the unique synergy between isometric exercises and the pursuit of supple joints, offering a path toward improved overall flexibility and joint well-being.

The Intricate Connection:

Understanding the intricate connection between isometric training, flexibility, and joint health lays the foundation for this exploration:

Isometrics and Muscle Elongation:

Explanation:

    1. Isometric exercises involve static contractions without joint movement.

    2. The sustained holds in isometrics contribute to muscle elongation, fostering flexibility.

Joint Stability Through Isometrics:

Explanation:

    1. Isometric holds promote joint stability by engaging surrounding muscles.

    2. This stability enhances joint health, providing a foundation for improved flexibility.

Strategic Isometric Holds for Flexibility:

Discover the strategic use of isometric holds to enhance flexibility:

Targeting Major Muscle Groups:

Guidance:

1. Identify major muscle groups associated with the desired flexibility improvement.

2. Design isometric holds that engage and elongate these muscles, promoting flexibility.

Incorporating Controlled Stretching:

Guidance:

1. Integrate controlled stretching within isometric holds.

2. This combination amplifies the stretching effect, contributing to increased flexibility.

Joint Health and Isometric Training:

Delve into how isometric training supports joint health:

Minimizing Impact on Joints:

Guidance:

1. Isometric exercises minimize impact on joints as there is no repetitive joint movement.

2. This gentle approach safeguards joint health, particularly beneficial for seniors.

Engaging Surrounding Muscles:

Guidance:

1. Isometric holds engage surrounding muscles that support and stabilize joints.

2. Enhanced muscle engagement contributes to overall joint health.

Specialized Isometric Exercises for Flexibility:
Explore specialized isometric exercises designed to target flexibility:

Isometric Hip Flexor Stretch:
Execution:
1. Assume a lunge position.
2. Lower the hips to deepen the stretch.
3. Hold the position for 20-30 seconds, focusing on elongating the hip flexors.

Wall Chest Opener Hold:
Execution:
1. Stand facing a wall.
2. Place one arm on the wall at shoulder height and turn away, feeling a stretch across the chest.
3. Hold for 15-20 seconds, emphasizing the chest opening.

Integrating Flexibility into Isometric Routines:

Learn how to seamlessly integrate flexibility into your isometric routines:

Warm-Up with Dynamic Stretches:

Guidance:

 1. Begin each session with dynamic stretches to prepare muscles for isometric holds.

 2. Dynamic stretching primes the muscles for enhanced flexibility during isometrics.

Cool Down with Isometric Stretches:

Guidance:

 1. Conclude workouts with isometric stretches.

 2. These stretches aid in muscle recovery and further contribute to flexibility gains.

Conclusion:

As we conclude Chapter 5, the interplay between isometric training, flexibility, and joint health comes to the forefront. The strategic use of isometrics not only elongates muscles for improved flexibility but also nurtures joint health, creating a harmonious balance. This chapter serves as a guide, illuminating the path toward supple joints and enhanced flexibility through the power of isometric training.

Key Takeaways:

- Isometric exercises contribute to muscle elongation, fostering flexibility.
- Strategic isometric holds target major muscle groups, promoting flexibility.

- Isometric training minimizes impact on joints, supporting overall joint health.
- Specialized isometric exercises, such as hip flexor stretches and chest openers, enhance flexibility.
- Seamlessly integrate flexibility into isometric routines with dynamic warm-ups and isometric stretches during cool-down.

Chapter 5
10-Minute Daily Routines for Maximum Impact
Creating Manageable and Consistent Exercise Habits

Introduction:

In Chapter 5 of "Isometric Strength for Seniors," we explore the transformative potential of short, consistent isometric routines. This chapter is dedicated to creating manageable and consistent exercise habits that maximize impact within just 10 minutes a day. Join us as we unravel the power of daily commitment and its profound effects on overall health and well-being.

The Essence of Consistency:

Understanding the essence of consistency lays the groundwork for this chapter:

Daily vs. Intermittent Exercise:

Explanation:

 1. Daily isometric routines establish a consistent exercise habit.

 2. This approach contrasts with intermittent or sporadic exercise patterns.

Cumulative Benefits of Daily Habits:

Explanation:

 1. Daily exercise accumulates benefits over time.

 2. The cumulative effect contributes to sustained improvements in strength, flexibility, and overall health.

Overcoming Time Constraints:

Addressing time constraints is key to making daily routines manageable:

The 10-Minute Solution:

Guidance:

1. A 10-minute daily routine is a feasible solution for busy schedules.

2. The manageable timeframe makes consistent exercise accessible to everyone.

Prioritizing Brief, Regular Sessions:

Guidance:

1. Prioritize short, regular sessions over lengthy, infrequent workouts.

2. Brief sessions ensure sustained engagement and adherence to the routine.

Crafting Your 10-Minute Routine:

Designing a personalized 10-minute isometric routine enhances its impact:

Targeting Key Areas:

Guidance:

1. Identify key areas for improvement, such as strength, flexibility, or joint health.

2. Tailor exercises to target these specific areas within the 10-minute timeframe.

Guidance:

1. Rotate the focus of your routine to address different aspects of fitness.

2. This rotation prevents monotony and ensures holistic benefits.

Sample 10-Minute Isometric Routine:

Explore a sample routine that showcases the diversity of exercises within a 10-minute timeframe:

Isometric Squat Holds (2 minutes):

Execution:

1. Stand with feet shoulder-width apart and lower into a squat position.

2. Hold the squat for 30 seconds, gradually increasing the duration.

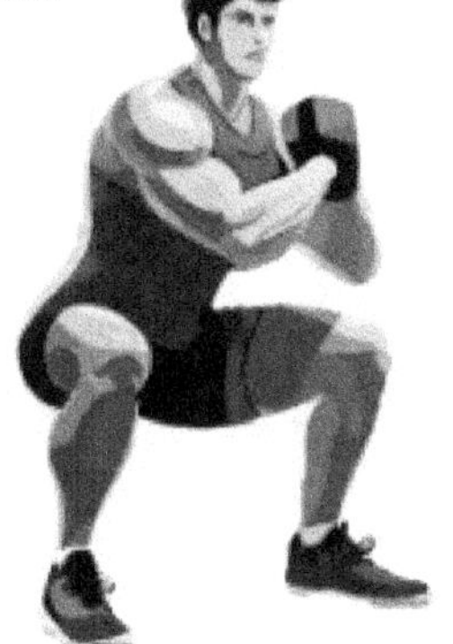

Wall Push-Up Holds (2 minutes):

Execution:

1. Perform push-ups against a wall, pausing midway for a static hold.

2. Hold for 30 seconds, focusing on engaging the chest and arms.

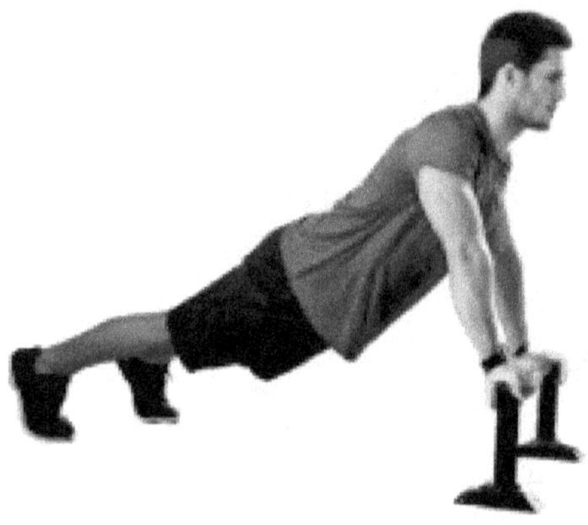

Dynamic Leg Raises (3 minutes):

Execution:

1. Lie on your back and lift one leg at a time, engaging the core.

2. Perform dynamic leg raises for 45 seconds per leg.

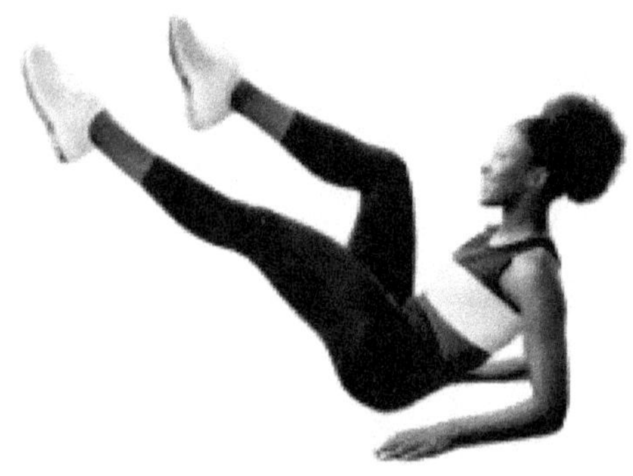

Seated Isometric Shoulder Press (2 minutes):

Execution:

1. Sit with a straight back and press your hands together overhead.

2. Hold the press for 30 seconds, feeling the engagement in the shoulders.

Making Consistency a Habit:

Turning daily routines into habits involves understanding the psychology of habit formation:

Set a Regular Schedule:

Guidance:

1. Establish a fixed time for your 10-minute routine each day.

2. Consistency in timing reinforces the habit.

Anchor Your Routine to Existing Habits:

Guidance:

1. Attach your routine to an existing habit, like morning coffee or evening TV time.

2. This anchoring technique integrates the routine seamlessly into your daily life.

Conclusion:

This chapter concludes with the recognition that 10 minutes a day can lead to remarkable transformations when embraced consistently. By crafting manageable and consistent exercise habits, you not only improve your physical health but also cultivate a positive and enduring lifestyle change.

Key Takeaways:

- Daily isometric routines offer cumulative benefits over time.
- A 10-minute daily routine is a manageable solution for busy schedules.
- Personalize your routine to target specific fitness goals within the 10-minute timeframe.

- Sample routines can include exercises targeting strength, flexibility, and joint health.
- Establish consistency by setting a regular schedule and anchoring your routine to existing habits.

Quick and Effective Isometric Workouts for Busy Schedules

Introduction:

In this Chapter of "Isometric Strength for Seniors," we dive into the realm of quick and effective isometric workouts tailored for busy schedules. This chapter is designed to provide step-by-step explanations for each exercise, ensuring that even in the midst of a hectic lifestyle, you can harness the benefits of isometric training efficiently.

The Essence of Quick Workouts:

Understanding the essence of quick workouts sets the tone for this chapter:

Time-Efficiency as a Priority:

Explanation:

1. Quick workouts prioritize time-efficiency.

2. They deliver maximum impact in a condensed timeframe, ideal for busy schedules.

Integration into Daily Routines:

Explanation:

1. Quick workouts seamlessly integrate into daily routines.

2. They serve as accessible and efficient bursts of physical activity.

Engage major muscle groups with this simple yet effective isometric exercise:

Execution:

1. Stand with your back against a wall and lower into a seated position, forming a 90-degree angle with your knees.

2. Hold the position for 1 minute, focusing on engaging your quadriceps and glutes.

3. Gradually increase the duration as your strength improves.

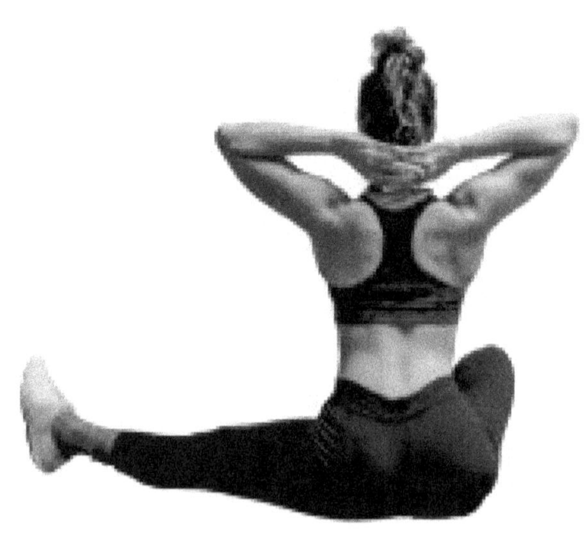

Strengthen your core and improve overall stability with plank holds:

Execution:

1. Assume a plank position on your hands or forearms, ensuring a straight line from head to heels.

2. Hold the plank for 30 seconds to 1 minute, engaging your core muscles.

3. Increase the duration gradually, maintaining proper form.

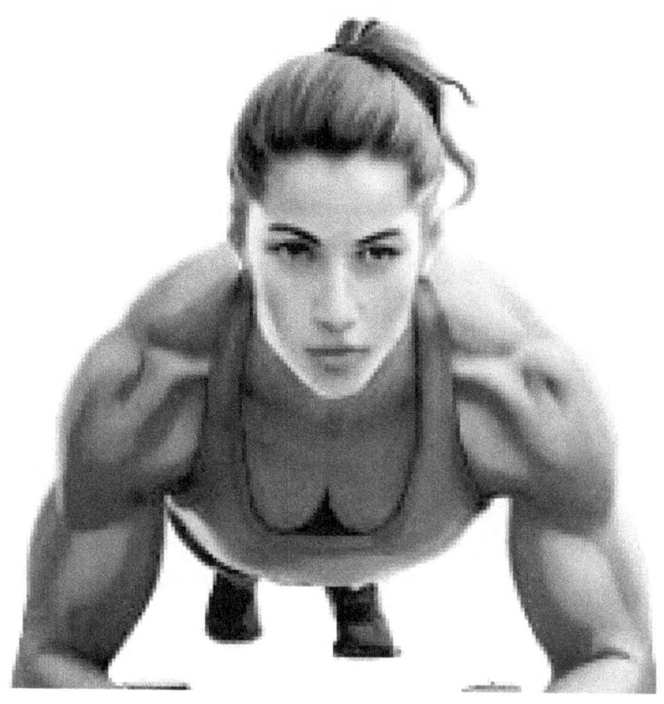

Target the upper body and chest with this variation of the classic push-up:

Execution:

1. Begin in a push-up position.

2. Lower halfway and hold the position for 30 seconds, emphasizing chest and arm engagement.

3. Gradually extend the duration as your strength develops.

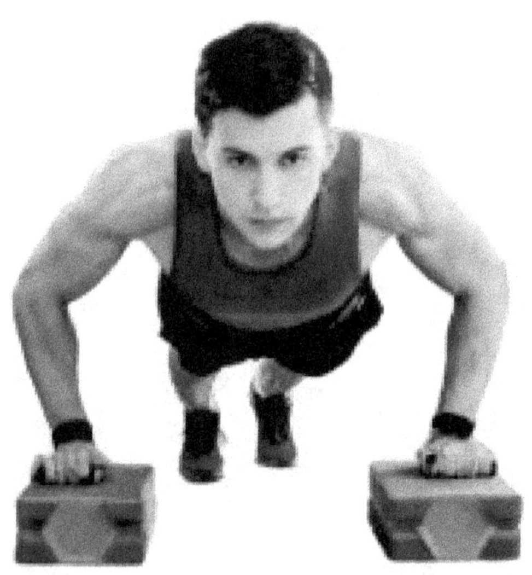

Focus on lower body strength with this seated variation:

Execution:

1. Sit on a stable chair with your back straight.

2. Press your legs together and hold the position for 30 seconds to 1 minute.

3. Feel the engagement in your thighs and glutes, adjusting intensity as needed.

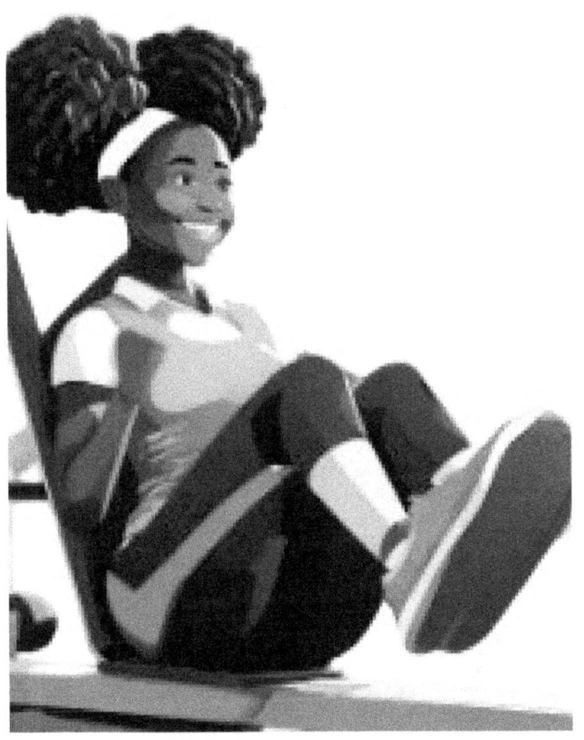

Target your arm muscles with this convenient and effective isometric exercise:

Execution:

1. Hold a light weight or resistance band in both hands, palms facing forward.

2. Curl the weight halfway and hold for 30 seconds, focusing on bicep engagement.

3. Gradually increase the duration as your strength improves.

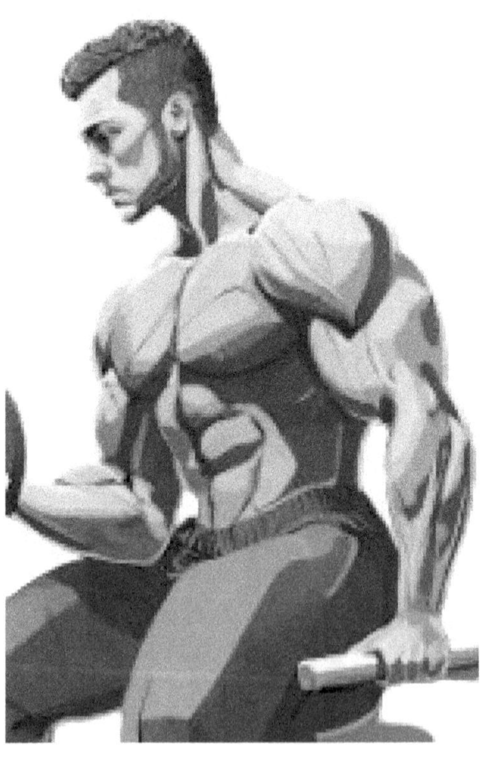

Incorporating Quick Workouts into Your Day:

Seamlessly integrate quick isometric workouts into your daily routine:

Morning Energizer:

Guidance:

1. Perform a quick wall sit or plank routine in the morning to kickstart your day.

2. These exercises boost energy levels and set a positive tone.

Desk Breaks:

Guidance:

1. Take short breaks during work hours for a quick isometric exercise.

2. Incorporate exercises like seated leg presses or bicep curls to refresh your mind and body.

Conclusion:

As the Chapter concludes, the emphasis on quick and effective isometric workouts for busy schedules remains clear. With step-by-step explanations for each exercise, you possess the tools to infuse moments of strength-building into even the most time-constrained days.

Key Takeaways:

- Quick workouts prioritize time-efficiency for busy schedules.
- Wall sit holds, plank holds, isometric push-ups, seated leg presses, and bicep curls are versatile exercises suitable for short routines.

- Gradually increase the duration and intensity of each exercise as your strength improves.
- Seamlessly integrate quick workouts into your daily routine for consistent benefits.

Chapter 6
Enhancing Overall Health with Isometric Strength
Cardiovascular Benefits of Isometric Training

Introduction:

In Chapter 6 of "Isometric Strength for Seniors," we delve into the multifaceted benefits of isometric training, with a particular focus on its impact on cardiovascular health. This chapter illuminates the ways in which isometric strength exercises contribute to enhanced overall well-being by positively influencing cardiovascular function.

Understanding Cardiovascular Benefits:

Establishing a foundation for the discussion, let's explore the fundamental cardiovascular benefits of isometric training:

Isometrics and Heart Health:

Explanation:

1. Isometric exercises require sustained muscle contractions.

2. These contractions elicit cardiovascular responses, contributing to heart health.

Blood Pressure Regulation:

Explanation:

1. Isometric training engages muscles, promoting efficient blood circulation.

2. Improved circulation assists in regulating blood pressure levels.

Cardiovascular Response during Isometrics:

Understanding how the cardiovascular system responds during isometric exercises lays the groundwork for this chapter:

Increased Heart Rate:

Explanation:

1. Isometric contractions demand increased oxygen delivery to active muscles.

2. The heart responds by elevating the heart rate, enhancing cardiovascular conditioning.

Enhanced Stroke Volume:

Explanation:

1. Isometrics lead to stronger, more forceful muscle contractions.

2. This increases stroke volume—the amount of blood pumped per heartbeat—improving overall cardiac efficiency.

Benefits for Seniors:

Explore how these cardiovascular benefits are particularly advantageous for the senior demographic:

Managing Hypertension:

Guidance:

1. Isometric training assists in managing hypertension, a common concern among seniors.

2. Regular isometric exercises contribute to maintaining healthy blood pressure levels.

Guidance:

1. Aging can impact cardiovascular function.

2. Isometric strength training becomes a proactive approach to promoting heart health as individuals age.

Sample Cardiovascular Isometric Routine:

Engage in a sample routine designed to specifically target cardiovascular health:

Dynamic Isometric Wall Push-Ups (3 minutes):

Execution:

1. Perform wall push-ups dynamically, adding a small bounce in each repetition.

2. Engages chest, shoulders, and arms while promoting cardiovascular response.

Isometric Squat Jumps (2 minutes):

Execution:

1. Perform isometric squats, adding explosive jumps during the hold.

2. Elevates heart rate and enhances cardiovascular conditioning.

Isometric Plank with Knee Taps (2 minutes):

Execution:

1. Hold a plank position and alternately tap your knees to the ground.

2. Introduces dynamic movement within isometric holds, stimulating cardiovascular response.

Incorporating Cardiovascular Isometrics into Your Routine:

Guidelines for seamlessly integrating cardiovascular isometrics into your overall routine:

Frequency and Duration:

Guidance:

1. Aim for at least three cardiovascular isometric sessions per week.

2. Each session may last 20-30 minutes, including warm-up and cool-down.

Progression and Adaptation:

Guidance:

1. Gradually increase the intensity and duration of cardiovascular isometric exercises.

2. Adapt the routine based on individual fitness levels and goals.

Conclusion:

As this Chapter concludes, the understanding of how isometric training positively influences cardiovascular health becomes a cornerstone for overall well-being. By embracing the cardiovascular benefits of isometric strength exercises, individuals, especially seniors, can foster a heart-healthy lifestyle.

Key Takeaways:

- Isometric training elicits cardiovascular responses, contributing to heart health.
- Improved blood circulation and regulated blood pressure are key cardiovascular benefits.

- Seniors can manage hypertension and promote heart health through regular isometric exercises.
- Sample routines, like dynamic wall push-ups and isometric squat jumps, can be integrated for cardiovascular benefits.
- Strategic incorporation of cardiovascular isometrics, following guidelines, becomes a proactive approach to overall health.

Stress Reduction and Mental Well-Being

Introduction:

In this chapter of "Isometric Strength for Seniors," we explore the profound impact of isometric training on stress reduction and mental well-being. This chapter delves into the interconnected relationship between physical exercise, particularly isometrics, and the enhancement of mental health.

The Mind-Body Connection:

Understanding the intricate link between the body and mind sets the stage for this exploration:

Holistic Health Approach:

Explanation:

    1. Physical exercise, including isometric training, has a direct impact on mental well-being.

    2. The mind-body connection forms the basis for a holistic approach to health.

Hormonal Regulation:

Explanation:

    1. Isometric exercises regulate the release of stress hormones.

    2. This hormonal balance contributes to a more stable and positive mental state.

Stress Reduction Mechanisms:

Uncover the specific mechanisms through which isometric training aids in stress reduction:

Cortisol Regulation:

Explanation:

1. Isometric exercises assist in regulating cortisol levels.

2. Cortisol, known as the stress hormone, is balanced, reducing overall stress.

Endorphin Release:

Explanation:

1. Isometric training triggers the release of endorphins, the body's natural mood lifters.

2. Increased endorphins contribute to a sense of well-being and stress relief.

Cognitive Benefits:

Explore the cognitive benefits that accompany stress reduction through isometric training:

Improved Focus and Concentration:

Guidance:

1. Regular isometric exercise enhances cognitive function.

2. Improved focus and concentration are natural byproducts of reduced stress.

Sleep Quality Enhancement:

Guidance:

1. Isometric training aids in relaxation, promoting better sleep quality.

2. Quality sleep is a cornerstone of mental well-being.

Mindful Isometric Practices:

Incorporate mindfulness into isometric exercises for enhanced stress reduction:

Mindful Breathing during Holds:

Guidance:

1. Practice mindful breathing during isometric holds.

2. Deep, intentional breaths enhance the relaxation response.

Visualization Techniques:

Guidance:

1. Incorporate positive visualization during isometric exercises.

2. Visualizing calm environments or personal achievements amplifies the stress-relieving effects.

Integrating Isometric Practices into Daily Life:

Guidelines for seamlessly integrating isometric practices into daily routines for ongoing mental well-being:

Micro-Breaks at Work:

Guidance:

1. Incorporate brief isometric exercises during work breaks.

2. Micro-breaks foster mental rejuvenation and stress relief.

Evening Stress-Relief Routine:

Guidance:

1. Establish an evening isometric routine as part of winding down.

2. Stress reduction practices contribute to a more restful night.

Conclusion:
As Chapter concludes, the understanding of how isometric training contributes to stress reduction and mental well-being becomes a valuable tool in the pursuit of holistic health. By embracing the interconnectedness of physical and mental health, individuals can cultivate a resilient and positive mindset through the practice of isometrics.

Key Takeaways:
- Isometric training plays a pivotal role in stress reduction and mental well-being.
- Hormonal regulation, including cortisol balance and endorphin release, contributes to stress relief.
- Cognitive benefits, such as improved focus and better sleep quality, accompany reduced stress.
- Mindful isometric practices enhance stress reduction through intentional breathing and visualization.
- Integrating isometric practices into daily routines becomes a sustainable approach to ongoing mental well-being.

Turn the page, armed with the knowledge that each isometric session not only strengthens the body but also nurtures the mind, fostering a resilient and positive outlook on life.

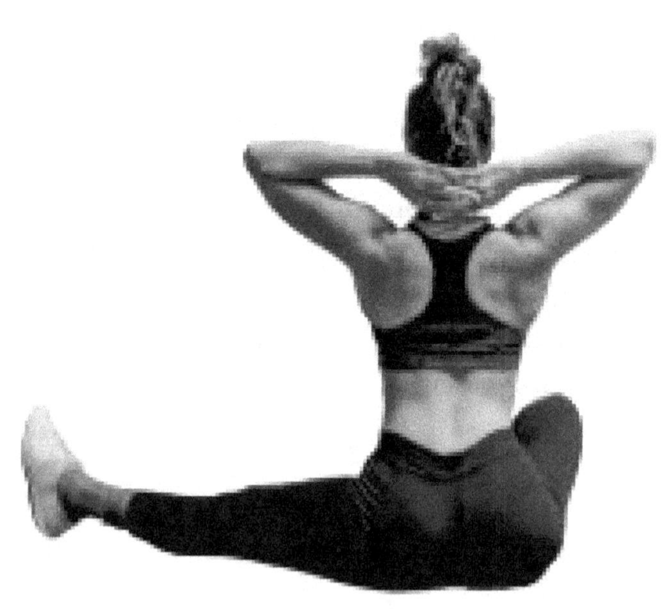

Chapter 7
Nutrition Tips for Supporting Isometric Training
Exploring Different Exercise Modalities

Introduction:

In Chapter 7 of "Isometric Strength for Seniors," we delve into the pivotal role of nutrition in supporting isometric training. This chapter underscores the importance of a well-balanced diet in senior fitness, elucidating how proper nutrition complements and enhances the benefits of isometric exercises.

Understanding the Senior Fitness Landscape:

Setting the context, let's explore the unique considerations of senior fitness:

Changing Nutritional Needs:

Explanation:

1. Aging brings changes in metabolism, nutrient absorption, and muscle maintenance.

2. Understanding these shifts is crucial for tailoring nutrition to support senior fitness.

Isometric Training and Nutrient Requirements:

Explanation:

1. Isometric exercises demand specific nutrients for muscle recovery and energy.

2. Tailoring nutrition to meet these demands optimizes the effectiveness of isometric training.

2 Essential Nutrients for Senior Fitness:

Explore the key nutrients that play a vital role in supporting isometric training for seniors:

Protein for Muscle Maintenance:

Guidance:

1. Adequate protein intake supports muscle maintenance and repair.
2. Include lean sources of protein like poultry, fish, beans, and dairy in your diet.

Calcium and Vitamin D for Bone Health:

Guidance:

1. Senior fitness places emphasis on bone health.
2. Ensure sufficient calcium and vitamin D intake through dairy, leafy greens, and sunlight exposure.

Hydration for Optimal Performance:

Highlight the significance of proper hydration in the context of isometric training:

Water Intake Recommendations:

Guidance:

1. Seniors should maintain consistent hydration.
2. Aim for at least 8 glasses of water daily, adjusting based on individual needs and activity levels.

Electrolyte Balance:

Guidance:

1. Isometric training may lead to electrolyte loss through sweat.

2. Include electrolyte-rich foods like bananas and oranges to restore balance.

The Role of Nutrient Timing:

Understanding when to fuel the body is crucial for optimizing isometric training benefits:

Pre-Workout Nutrition:

Guidance:

1. Consume a balanced meal with carbohydrates and protein 1-2 hours before isometric sessions.
2. Provides sustained energy for the workout.

Post-Workout Recovery:

Guidance:

1. Include a post-workout meal or snack with protein and carbohydrates within 30-60 minutes.
2. Supports muscle recovery and replenishes glycogen stores.

Addressing Specific Dietary Concerns:

Tailor nutrition recommendations to address specific dietary concerns often encountered by seniors:

Managing Chronic Conditions:

Guidance:

1. Consider dietary modifications to manage conditions like diabetes or hypertension.
2. Work with a healthcare professional or nutritionist for personalized guidance.

Guidance:

1. Seniors may be at risk for certain nutrient deficiencies.

2. Regular health check-ups can help identify and address these deficiencies.

Conclusion:

The integral relationship between nutrition and senior fitness becomes apparent. By understanding the evolving nutritional needs of seniors and tailoring dietary choices to support isometric training, individuals can maximize the benefits of their fitness journey.

Key Takeaways:

- Nutrition plays a pivotal role in supporting the effectiveness of isometric training for seniors.
- Essential nutrients like protein, calcium, and vitamin D are crucial for muscle and bone health.
- Proper hydration and electrolyte balance are essential components of senior fitness nutrition.
- Strategic nutrient timing, both pre and post-workout, enhances overall performance and recovery.
- Addressing specific dietary concerns ensures a holistic approach to senior fitness nutrition.

Foods That Aid Muscle Strength and Recovery

Introduction:

In Chapter 8 of "Isometric Strength for Seniors," we dive into the world of nutrition tailored specifically to support muscle strength and recovery. This chapter focuses on the role of food in optimizing the benefits of isometric training, providing seniors with a comprehensive guide to nourishing their bodies for sustained strength and efficient recovery.

The Synergy of Nutrition and Isometric Training:

Understanding the interconnected relationship between nutrition and isometric training forms the basis for this exploration:

Muscle Fueling:

Explanation:

1. Isometric training demands energy for sustained muscle contractions.

2. Optimal nutrition ensures sufficient fuel for workouts and recovery.

Post-Exercise Repair:

Explanation:

1. Effective recovery relies on the availability of nutrients post-exercise.

2. Specific foods aid in muscle repair and regeneration after isometric sessions.

Protein-Rich Foods for Muscle Maintenance:

Explore the essential role of protein in supporting muscle strength and recovery:

Lean Protein Sources:

Guidance:

1. Include lean proteins such as chicken, turkey, fish, and plant-based options like beans and lentils.

2. Supports muscle maintenance and repair without excess saturated fats.

Greek Yogurt and Cottage Cheese:

Guidance:

1. High in protein and rich in essential amino acids.

2. Ideal as a snack or part of a post-workout meal for muscle recovery.

Nutrient-Dense Carbohydrates:

Highlight the importance of carbohydrates in providing energy for isometric training:

Whole Grains:

Guidance:

1. Choose whole grains like brown rice, quinoa, and oats.

2. Complex carbohydrates sustain energy levels for prolonged isometric sessions.

Fruits and Vegetables:

Guidance:

1. Colorful fruits and vegetables provide vitamins, minerals, and antioxidants.

2. Support overall health and contribute to sustained energy.

Healthy Fats for Recovery:

Understand the role of healthy fats in promoting recovery and overall well-being:

Avocado and Nuts:

Guidance:

1. Rich in monounsaturated fats and essential nutrients.

2. Contribute to post-exercise recovery and provide sustained energy.

Fatty Fish:

Guidance:

1. Salmon, mackerel, and sardines are high in omega-3 fatty acids.

2. Anti-inflammatory properties aid in muscle recovery and joint health.

Hydration for Efficient Recovery:

Emphasize the importance of hydration in the muscle recovery process:

Water and Electrolytes:

Guidance:

1. Stay well-hydrated throughout the day.

2. Replenish electrolytes with natural sources like coconut water or consume sports drinks if needed.

Timing and Portion Control:

Offer guidelines on when and how much to eat for optimal muscle support:

Pre-Workout Snacks:

Guidance:

1. Consume a balanced snack with a mix of carbohydrates and protein 1-2 hours before isometric training.

2. Provides sustained energy and prepares the body for exercise.

Post-Workout Meals:

Guidance:

1. Prioritize a post-workout meal or snack rich in protein and carbohydrates within 30-60 minutes.

2. Aids in muscle recovery and replenishes glycogen stores.

Conclusion:

As the Chapter concludes, the significance of selecting nutrient-dense foods for muscle strength and recovery becomes evident. By incorporating a variety of protein sources, complex carbohydrates, healthy fats, and staying well-hydrated, seniors can optimize the benefits of isometric training and foster a resilient and nourished body.

Key Takeaways:

- Protein-rich foods support muscle maintenance and repair.
- Nutrient-dense carbohydrates provide sustained energy for isometric training.
- Healthy fats contribute to post-exercise recovery and overall well-being.
- Hydration is crucial for efficient muscle recovery.

Chapter 8
Overcoming Common Challenges
Dealing with Joint Pain and Arthritis

Introduction:

In Chapter 8 of "Isometric Strength for Seniors," we address a prevalent concern among older adults—joint pain and arthritis. This chapter is dedicated to providing practical insights and strategies to overcome these challenges, ensuring that individuals can engage in isometric training with confidence and ease.

Understanding Joint Pain and Arthritis:

Lay the groundwork by elucidating the common challenges seniors face with joint pain and arthritis:

Age-Related Joint Changes:

Explanation:

    1. Aging often brings degenerative changes to joints.

    2. Cartilage wears down, leading to joint discomfort and stiffness.

Impact on Mobility:

Explanation:

    1. Joint pain and arthritis can hinder mobility.

    2. Limitations in movement affect daily activities and exercise engagement.

The Role of Isometric Training in Joint Health:

Highlight the potential benefits of isometric training in managing joint pain:

Guidance:

1. Isometric exercises are low-impact, placing minimal stress on joints.

2. Ideal for individuals with joint pain seeking a gentle yet effective workout.

Guidance:

1. Strengthening surrounding muscles provides better joint support.

2. Isometric training aids in building muscle strength without excessive joint movement.

Tailoring Isometric Exercises for Joint Health:

Provide specific strategies to adapt isometric exercises for individuals with joint pain:

Guidance:

1. Adjust the range of motion in isometric exercises.

2. Focus on the pain-free range to prevent exacerbating joint discomfort.

Guidance:

1. Incorporate seated variations for exercises like leg lifts or bicep curls.

2. Reduces stress on weight-bearing joints.

Incorporating Joint-Friendly Nutritional Choices:

Explore dietary considerations to complement isometric training for joint health:

Omega-3 Fatty Acids:

Guidance:

1. Include foods rich in omega-3s like fatty fish, flaxseeds, and walnuts.

2. Known for their anti-inflammatory properties, supporting joint health.

Collagen-Rich Foods:

Guidance:

1. Collagen supports joint and connective tissue health.

2. Incorporate collagen-rich foods such as bone broth, chicken, and fish.

Seeking Professional Guidance:

Encourage readers to consult healthcare professionals for personalized advice:

Physical Therapist Consultation:

Guidance:

1. Seek guidance from a physical therapist.

2. Customized exercises and recommendations tailored to individual needs.

Nutritionist Collaboration:

Guidance:

1. Collaborate with a nutritionist for dietary advice.

2. Tailor nutritional choices to support joint health and overall well-being.

The Power of Gradual Progression:

Emphasize the importance of gradual progression in isometric training:

Slow and Controlled Movements:

Guidance:

1. Emphasize slow and controlled movements in isometric exercises.

2. Reduces the risk of sudden joint strain.

Listening to Your Body:

Guidance:

1. Pay attention to joint sensations during and after exercises.

2. Modify or pause activities if discomfort arises.

Conclusion:

As this Chapter concludes, the overarching theme is empowerment, empowering individuals to overcome common challenges associated with joint pain and arthritis. By understanding the benefits of isometric training, tailoring exercises, embracing joint-friendly nutrition, seeking professional guidance, and progressing at a comfortable pace, seniors can engage in a fulfilling and joint-friendly fitness journey.

Key Takeaways:

- Isometric training offers a low-impact option for individuals with joint pain and arthritis.
- Tailor isometric exercises with range-of-motion modifications and seated variations.

- Consider incorporating joint-friendly nutrients like omega-3 fatty acids and collagen.
- Collaboration with healthcare professionals enhances personalized guidance.
- Gradual progression and attentive listening to the body are key principles for joint health.

Modifications for Seniors with Limited Mobility

Introduction:

In this Chapter of "Isometric Strength for Seniors," we address the unique needs of individuals with limited mobility. This chapter is dedicated to providing thoughtful modifications for isometric exercises, ensuring that seniors with mobility challenges can participate in the benefits of isometric training with comfort and confidence.

Understanding Limited Mobility:

Begin by acknowledging the challenges faced by seniors with limited mobility:

Mobility Barriers:

Explanation:

    1. Limited mobility may stem from various factors, including joint issues, injuries, or chronic conditions.

    2. Identifying and understanding specific mobility barriers is crucial for tailored modifications.

Importance of Inclusivity:

Explanation:

    1. An inclusive approach ensures that isometric training is accessible to individuals with varying degrees of mobility.

    2. Modifying exercises allows for a personalized and adaptable fitness experience.

Seated Isometric Exercises:

Introduce modifications that can be performed from a seated position:

Seated Leg Raises:

Guidance:

1. Sit comfortably in a chair with feet flat on the floor.

2. Lift one leg at a time, engaging the muscles without putting strain on joints.

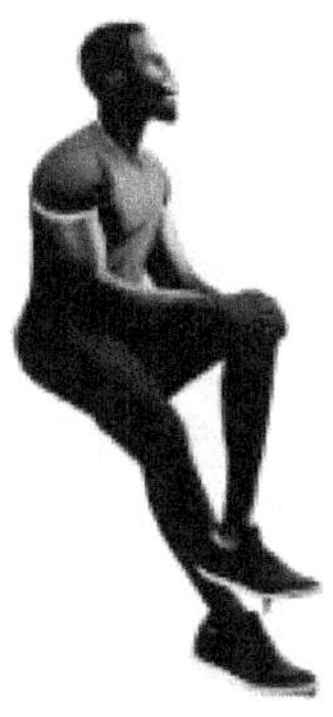

Seated Chest Press:

Guidance:

1. Use resistance bands or lightweights while seated.

2. Mimic a chest press motion, focusing on controlled movements.

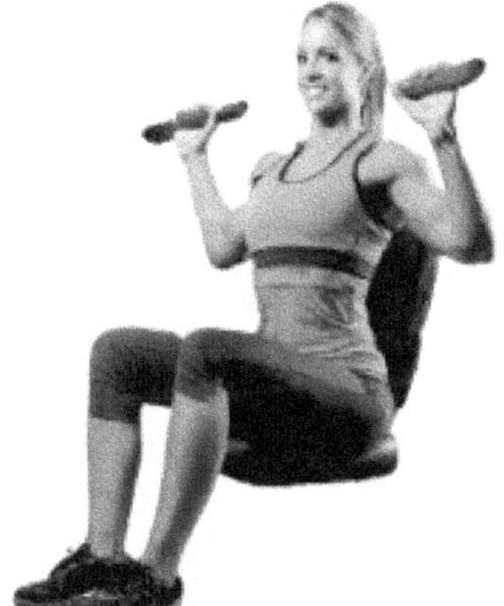

Gentle Range-of-Motion Exercises:

Highlight modifications emphasizing gentle range-of-motion:

Arm Circles:

Guidance:

1. Stand or sit with arms extended.

2. Perform slow and controlled circular motions, promoting flexibility without excessive strain.

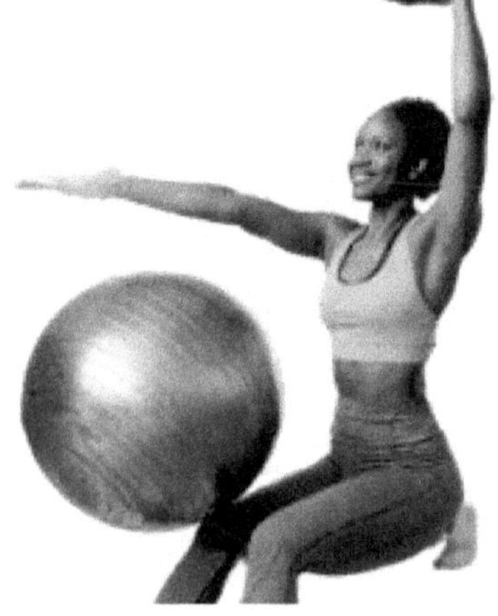

Neck Tilts and Turns:

Guidance:

1. While seated, gently tilt and turn the neck.

2. Enhances mobility in the cervical spine without rigorous movements.

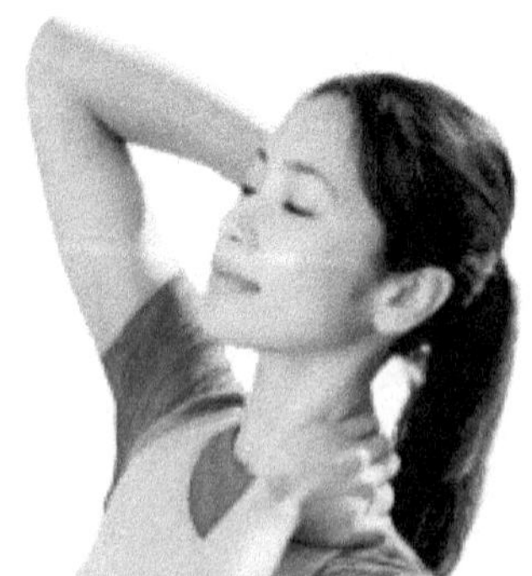

Adaptations for Standing Exercises:

Explore modifications for standing exercises, considering balance and stability:

Wall-Assisted Squats:

Guidance:

1. Stand with the back against a wall for support.

2. Perform partial squats, focusing on form and engaging leg muscles.

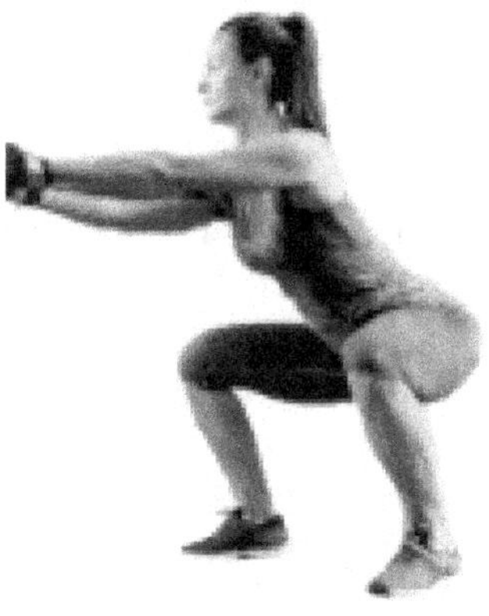

Wall Push-Ups:

Guidance:

1. Face a wall with hands placed at shoulder height.

2. Execute push-ups against the wall, adjusting intensity based on comfort.

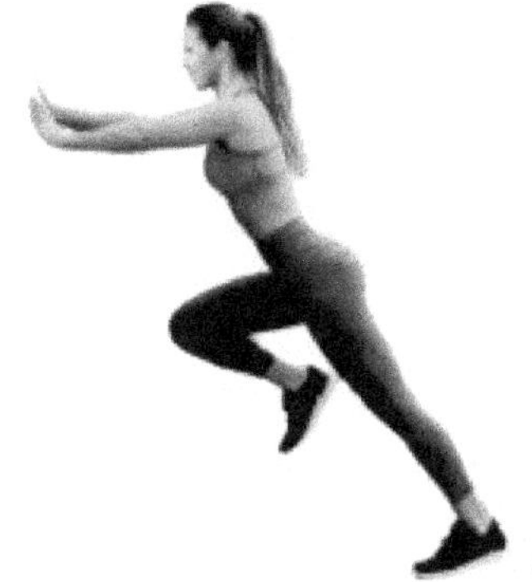

Incorporating Assistive Devices:

Discuss the integration of assistive devices for enhanced stability:

Chair Stability:

Guidance:

1. Place a sturdy chair nearby for support.

2. Provides stability during exercises, fostering confidence and safety.

Resistance Bands with Handles:

Guidance:

1. Utilize resistance bands with handles for seated or standing exercises.

2. Adds resistance without the need for heavy weights.

Individualized Modifications:

Empower seniors to customize modifications based on their unique needs:

Personalized Adaptations:

Guidance:

1. Encourage experimentation with movements to find comfortable variations.

2. Emphasize the importance of listening to the body and adapting as needed.

Chapter 9
Staying Motivated and Consistent
Setting Realistic Goals

Introduction:

In Chapter 9 of "Isometric Strength for Seniors," we explore the crucial aspects of staying motivated and consistent in isometric training. This chapter is dedicated to providing guidance on setting realistic goals, celebrating achievements, and maintaining a positive mindset throughout the fitness journey.

The Importance of Motivation and Consistency:

Establish the significance of maintaining motivation and consistency in isometric training:

Long-Term Benefits:

Explanation:

1. Consistent isometric training leads to long-term health and fitness benefits.

2. Regular practice enhances strength, flexibility, and overall well-being.

Building Habits:

Explanation:

1. Consistency builds habits, making isometric training an integral part of daily life.

2. Establishing a routine contributes to sustained progress.

Setting Realistic Goals:

Guide readers on the importance of setting achievable and meaningful goals:

Specificity in Goals:

Guidance:

1. Define specific isometric training goals, such as improving a particular exercise or increasing hold durations.
2. Specific goals provide clarity and direction.

Gradual Progression:

Guidance:

1. Set goals that allow for gradual progression.
2. Incremental improvements contribute to a sense of achievement and motivation.

Celebrating Achievements and Progress

Explore strategies for acknowledging and celebrating milestones:

Regular Progress Assessments:

Guidance:

1. Conduct regular assessments to track progress.

2. Celebrate improvements in strength, endurance, and overall performance.

Setting Milestone Rewards:

Guidance:

1. Establish milestone rewards for reaching specific goals.

2. Rewards could be a treat, a small purchase, or a moment of relaxation.

Embracing Positive Reinforcement:

Encourage the use of positive reinforcement for continued motivation:

Positive Self-Talk:

Guidance:

1. Cultivate a positive internal dialogue.

2. Replace self-doubt with affirmations to foster a constructive mindset.

External Encouragement:

Guidance:

1. Seek support from friends, family, or workout buddies.

2. External encouragement enhances motivation and accountability.

Overcoming Setbacks:

Address the inevitability of setbacks and provide strategies for resilience:

Learning from Setbacks:

Guidance:

1. View setbacks as opportunities for learning.
2. Analyze challenges and adapt goals accordingly.

Adjusting Expectations:

Guidance:

1. Be flexible in adjusting expectations.
2. Recognize that the fitness journey may have fluctuations, and that's normal.

Creating a Supportive Environment:

Highlight the importance of a positive and supportive environment:

Designing a Home Workout Space:

Guidance:

1. Create a dedicated and inviting space for isometric training at home.
2. A welcoming environment enhances motivation.

Joining Fitness Communities:

Guidance:

1. Connect with online or local fitness communities.
2. Sharing experiences and tips creates a sense of community support.

Chapter 10
Frequently Asked Questions
Addressing Common Concerns and Misconceptions

Introduction:

In the final chapter of "Isometric Strength for Seniors," we address a spectrum of frequently asked questions, aiming to provide clarity, dispel misconceptions, and address common concerns that may arise during the isometric training journey.

The Importance of Addressing FAQs:

Establish the significance of this chapter in providing comprehensive information and support:

Easing Apprehensions:

Explanation:

1. Frequently asked questions address common concerns, easing apprehensions that readers may have.

2. Clarity promotes confidence and commitment to the isometric training program.

Dismissing Misconceptions:

Explanation:

1. Addressing misconceptions ensures that readers have accurate information about isometric training.

2. Dismissing myths fosters a more informed and effective fitness journey.

Addressing Common Concerns:

Explore questions related to potential concerns that may arise during isometric training:

Is Isometric Training Safe for Seniors?

Answer:

1. Yes, isometric training is generally safe for seniors.

2. It is low-impact and can be tailored to individual fitness levels. Consultation with a healthcare professional is advisable for those with pre-existing conditions.

How Often Should Isometric Exercises Be Done?

Answer:

1. Frequency varies but starting with 2-3 sessions per week is recommended.

2. Consistency is key; gradually increase intensity and duration as comfort and strength improve.

Dispelling Misconceptions:

Address common misconceptions about isometric training:

Is Isometric Training Only for Building Muscle?

Answer:

1. While isometric training builds muscle strength, it also improves flexibility, joint health, and overall functional fitness.

2. It offers a holistic approach to senior wellness.

Answer:

1. Isometric exercises are low-impact and can be adapted for joint health.

2. Proper form, gradual progression, and modifications for individuals with joint concerns contribute to a joint-friendly approach.

Practical Tips and Advice:

Provide additional tips to enhance the isometric training experience:

Listening to the Body:

Advice:

1. Pay attention to how the body responds during and after exercises.

2. Modify intensity or exercises as needed to ensure comfort and safety.

Seeking Professional Guidance:

Advice:

1. Consult with healthcare professionals, especially for those with existing health conditions.

2. Physical therapists and nutritionists can offer personalized advice for an optimal fitness journey.

Encouragement for the Journey Ahead:

Conclude the chapter by offering encouragement and motivation:

Embracing Progress Over Perfection:

Encouragement:

1. Celebrate small victories and gradual progress.

2. Consistency and effort contribute to long-term success.

A Lifelong Journey to Wellness:

Encouragement:

1. Isometric training is part of a lifelong journey to wellness.

2. Embrace the journey with enthusiasm, knowing that each step contributes to improved health and vitality.

Conclusion:

As the chapter concludes, the compilation of frequently asked questions serves as a valuable resource for readers embarking on their isometric training journey. By addressing concerns, dispelling misconceptions, and providing practical tips, this chapter aims to empower seniors with the knowledge needed for a successful and enjoyable fitness experience.

Key Takeaways:

- Frequently asked questions provide clarity and address common concerns.
- Accurate information dispels misconceptions about isometric training.

- Listening to the body and seeking professional guidance contribute to a safe and effective fitness journey.
- Progress is celebrated over perfection, fostering a positive mindset.
- Isometric training is a lifelong journey to wellness, promoting sustained health and vitality.